FIFTH DISEASE

STEPS TO DEALING WITH FIFTH DISEASE

DR. J. SIMON

Contents

INTRODUCTION

Erythema infectiosum, also referred to as Fifth Disease, is a frequent childhood ailment brought on by the parvovirus B19. This viral infection, which is named after the fifth place in a historical categorization of pediatric rashes, mainly affects youngsters, however it can strike people at any age. Fifth Disease is characterized by a characteristic "slapped cheek" rash and, in certain cases, joint discomfort, even though it is often moderate. Let's examine the salient features of this contagious illness.

CHAPTER ONE

A Synopsis of Parvovirus B19

A tiny single-stranded DNA virus, parvovirus B19 is a member of the Parvoviridae family. It is the cause of erythema infectiosum, sometimes known as the Fifth Disease. Human erythroid progenitor cells, which are the precursors of red blood cells, are the cells that this virus prefers to infect. The primary means of transmission for the highly contagious parvovirus B19 is respiratory droplets.

Apart from producing Fifth Disease, arthropathy, or inflammation of the joints, and severe anemia, especially in those with underlying hemolytic diseases, are other clinical problems linked to

Parvovirus B19. It is noteworthy that the majority of Parvovirus B19 infections are minor and self-limiting, and that symptoms usually go away on their own without the need for special medical attention.

Term Uses and Historical Background

The Fifth Disease is referred to by a number of names that reflect its unique symptoms and historical background. Among the popular names are:

The infectious erythema

This is the medical term for Fifth Disease, and it's frequently used to refer to the infection's distinctive rash.

Smack-Cheek Illness:

This rash's unique "slapped cheek" appearance which resembles a reddish, slapped spot on the face is the source of its name.

Infection with Parvovirus B19:

This term highlights the virus-caused genesis of the disease and refers to Parvovirus B19, the causative virus.

The B19 human parvovirus disease:

Like its predecessor, this term highlights the particular virus that causes Fifth Disease.

The Fifth Illness

Based on past classifications of childhood rashes, when it was listed as the fifth ailment, the term "Fifth Disease" was coined. The other four were Duke's illness, rubella (German measles), scarlet fever, and measles.

Being the "fifth" on the list of typical childhood rashes in historical context is a reference to how these illnesses were formerly categorized. Knowing these names contributes to understanding the different facets and views that the illness has garnered over time.

Knowledge of the Fifth Illness

Erythema infectiosum, often known as Fifth Disease, is a viral infection brought on by the human parvovirus B19. Although it affects people of all ages, children are the ones who are most affected. The infection can be easily identified by its characteristic "slapped cheek" rash. Here are some important Fifth Disease concepts to comprehend:

Parvovirus B19: Parvovirus B19 is a tiny, single-stranded DNA virus that causes Fifth Disease. Respiratory droplets are how it spreads and is very contagious.

Respiratory Droplets: When an infected individual coughs or sneezes, the virus is mainly spread through respiratory droplets. Additionally, it can spread via contact with infected surfaces and by blood.

The rash known as "slapped cheek rash" is characterized by redness on both cheeks that gives the impression of being "slapped." A lacy red rash then appears over the arms, legs, and trunk.

temperature: A low temperature, headache, and weariness are common symptoms.

Joint Pain: More prevalent in adults, joint pain can be a symptom and last for a while.

Time of Incubation:

Fifth Disease typically takes 4 to 14 days to incubate after viral introduction.

Contagious Time Frame:

Before the rash appears, a person with Fifth Disease is most contagious. After the rash develops, there is far less chance of infection.

At-risk demographics

Although anyone can get the Fifth Disease, school-age children are the ones who get it most frequently. Those with compromised immune systems and expectant mothers may be more susceptible to difficulties.

Problems:

Most cases of Fifth Disease are minor and self-limiting. But occasionally, it can cause problems like arthropathy, or joint discomfort, and it can put particular groups at danger, such expectant mothers.

Clinical symptoms are frequently used to make the diagnosis, which is then verified by blood testing to look for antibodies or the presence of the virus.

Therapy:

Fifth Disease does not have a particular antiviral treatment. It is customary to advise symptomatic treatment, such as rest and over-the-counter painkillers.

Avoidance:

Avoiding contact with sick people and maintaining proper hygiene, such as frequent hand washing, can help stop the virus from spreading.

Considerations for Pregnancy:

If a pregnant woman contracts the Fifth Disease, she should visit a doctor since the developing fetus may be at risk. In these situations, medical supervision and monitoring are essential.

Even though Fifth Disease is usually not severe, it's nevertheless vital to recognize its signs, particularly in some cultures. It is crucial to seek medical guidance for an accurate diagnosis and course of treatment, especially for expectant mothers or people with underlying medical issues.

Erythema infectiosum, another name for fifth illness, is a viral infection brought on by parvovirus B19. It mainly affects kids, though it can happen to adults as well. A red rash on the face that resembles slapped cheeks is the hallmark symptom of fifth illness. The following are the symptoms and indicators of the fifth disease:

Rash on the Slapped Cheek:

A characteristic facial rash that gives the cheeks a flushed or "slapped" look is one of the telltale symptoms. Often, this is the first symptom that is apparent.

Body Rash with Lacy Pattern:

A lacy or net-like rash on the torso and limbs may appear after the facial rash. Over several weeks, this rash, which is usually red or pink, may appear and go.

Mild fever:

Many people with fifth illness have a low-grade fever, typically not going above 102°F (38.9°C). There are frequently other cold-like symptoms that accompany the fever.

Headache:

Headaches are one of the symptoms that some people may have of the fifth disease.

Throat Pain:

There may be a slight sore throat or pain in the throat that feels similar to the signs of a common cold.

Weary:

Although they are usually moderate, fatigue and a general sense of malaise might accompany the sickness.

It's crucial to remember that not everyone with a parvovirus B19 infection will experience symptoms; in fact, some people may only experience very minor ones. Furthermore, fifth disease is communicable in its early phases, frequently prior to the development of the recognizable rash. The person is usually no longer contagious once the rash appears.

It is best to seek medical assistance for a clear diagnosis and guidance on managing symptoms if someone is suspected of having fifth illness, particularly if they are pregnant or have a weakened immune system.

Identification and Assessment

Erythema infectiosum is a fifth illness that is frequently diagnosed based on clinical symptoms and physical examination. Laboratory testing, however, may occasionally be used by medical professionals to validate the diagnosis or determine the infection's stage. The following are typical techniques for identifying and evaluating the fifth disease:

Clinical Evaluation:

Medical professionals frequently identify fifth disease based on defining symptoms, particularly the development of a lacy rash over the trunk and limbs and a "slapped cheek" rash on the face. In most cases, the characteristic rash is adequate for diagnosis.

Blood Examinations:

Blood tests to identify particular antibodies or the presence of the parvovirus B19 may be carried out if further confirmation is required or if difficulties arise. Usually, two kinds of antibodies are examined:

IgM antibodies: These signify an infection that is either recent or ongoing.

IgG antibodies: These signify immunity or a previous infection.

PCR test, or polymerase chain reaction:

A PCR test may be utilized in some circumstances to identify the parvovirus B19's genetic makeup. When diagnosing acute infections, particularly in immunocompromised persons, this test can be useful.

Examining for any complication

If complications are thought to have resulted from the fifth disease, further testing may be carried out. For instance, joint fluid analysis testing may be carried out on those who have arthritis or joint pain.

CHAPTER TWO

It's crucial to remember that fifth disease is typically a mild, self-limiting sickness for which testing may not be required. However, in certain circumstances, such as during pregnancy or in people with compromised immune systems, testing might be advised.

It is important to see a healthcare provider for a proper diagnosis and suitable treatment if someone thinks they may have fifth illness or if there are concerns about complications. People who are immune system compromised or who are pregnant should consult a doctor right once.

Erythema infectiosum, often known as fifth illness, is usually a moderate viral infection that goes away on its own and doesn't always need medical attention. Nonetheless, a few strategies can aid in the management of the infection's symptoms and effects. The following are methods of treating the fifth disease:

Symptomatic Management:

Antiviral drugs are not necessary in the majority of fifth illness cases, since they resolve on their own. In order to manage symptoms like fever, headache, and joint discomfort, over-the-counter painkillers like acetaminophen or ibuprofen may be used.

Rest and Drinking Water:

It's imperative to get enough sleep and drink enough water to help the body's natural defense mechanism. People suffering with the fifth disease should be encouraged to rest and be well-hydrated by consuming enough of fluids, especially children.

Steer clear of aspirin:

It is crucial to refrain from administering aspirin to those who have fifth disease, particularly children. When used in conjunction with viral illnesses like as fifth disease, aspirin use has been linked to a higher chance of developing Reye's syndrome, an uncommon but dangerous illness.

Even though they are uncommon, people with fifth illness may have joint pain or swelling, especially in adults. In some situations, medical professionals could suggest extra steps or drugs to treat joint discomfort.

Handling Pregnancy:

It is imperative that a pregnant woman sees a healthcare professional if she gets symptoms or is exposed to the fifth disease. To determine the risk of complications, monitoring and additional assessment may be necessary in some circumstances. This is particularly true if there are worries about the effects on the growing fetus.

It's crucial to remember that the fifth disease is most infectious prior to the development of the recognizable rash. The person is usually no longer contagious once the rash appears. Consequently, people who exhibit fifth disease symptoms ought to take preventative measures to stop the virus from spreading, particularly in environments where there is intimate contact with expectant mothers or people who have compromised immune systems.

When in doubt or worried about potential problems, people should consult a physician for an appropriate assessment and direction.

Prevention and Contagion

Spread:

The fifth sickness, which is brought on by the parvovirus B19, is communicable and can be contracted by touching contaminated surfaces or respiratory droplets. Since the contagious period usually starts before symptoms appear, complete prevention of transmission is difficult. The principal means of communication consists of:

Transpiratory Transmission:

When an infected individual coughs or sneezes, respiratory droplets are frequently released into the air, spreading the virus. People who are around an infected individual may breathe in these droplets and become infected.

Direct Communication:

The virus can also spread by direct contact with saliva or respiratory secretions from an infected individual. Activities such as sharing utensils or kissing can cause this.

Polluted Surfaces:

The virus has a limited time of survival on surfaces. An infection may result from touching the mouth, nose, or eyes after coming into contact with surfaces tainted with respiratory secretions.

Avoidance:

By limiting exposure and maintaining proper cleanliness, the fifth disease can be stopped from spreading. The following are precautions to take:

Hand Sanitization:

Hand washing with soap and water on a regular basis is essential to stopping the virus from spreading. In the absence of soap and water, one can use hand sanitizers with alcohol base.

Breathing Hygiene:

Urge people to maintain proper respiratory hygiene by teaching them to cover their mouth and nose when they cough or sneeze by using an elbow or tissue. It's crucial to dispose of tissues properly and wash your hands very away.

Steer clear of close contact:

Avoid intimate contact, particularly with those who show signs of the fifth sickness. This is especially crucial for those who have never had the virus before, those with weakened immune systems, and expectant mothers.

Seclusion During the Spreading Phase:

Those who exhibit fifth illness symptoms ought to be aware of when the virus is communicable and take preventative measures to keep it from spreading. This entails abstaining from work or school until the infectious phase has ended.

Awareness of Pregnancy:

Women who are expecting should exercise caution and keep their distance from anyone exhibiting symptoms of the fifth disease. It is advised to seek medical attention as soon as possible if there is a possibility of exposure.

Cleaning of the Environment:

Keeping frequently touched surfaces clean and sterilised on a regular basis can help lower the risk of transmission, particularly in shared environments.

It's crucial to remember that although taking precautions can lower the chance of transmission, it might not be able to stop the virus from spreading completely, particularly in situations where there is close contact. In particular, for vulnerable populations, prompt medical attention and adherence to preventative measures are essential for managing the burden of fifth disease.

All ages can be affected by the fifth disease, erythema infectiosum, however some populations may be more susceptible to consequences or more severe symptoms. Among these populations are:

Kids:

Children are most commonly affected by fifth illness, especially those under the age of five. Children frequently have minimal symptoms or show no signs at all. across the other hand, they are more prone to get lacy rash across the body and the recognizable "slapped cheek" rash.

Expectant Mothers:

There is a higher chance of fifth illness problems in expectant mothers. A developing fetus may be at danger from infection during pregnancy, which could result in serious anemia or other issues. If a pregnant woman is exposed to the virus or experiences symptoms, she must visit a doctor.

People with Deflated Immune Systems:

People with compromised immune systems, like those with HIV/AIDS or undergoing chemotherapy, may be more vulnerable to fifth disease complications. Immunocompromised people may experience severe anemia as well as other problems.

People Affected by Hemolytic Disorders:

People who already suffer from hemolytic illnesses, like sickle cell anemia, may be more vulnerable to consequences from fifth disease, which can include severe anemia.

Healthcare Professionals:

Healthcare professionals should take protective measures to avoid exposure when they are in close proximity to patients who may be more susceptible to consequences, such as immunocompromised patients or pregnant women.

Daycare and School Environments:

Fifth illness is contagious, thus settings like schools and daycares might experience outbreaks. There is a higher chance that children in these settings will come into contact with the virus.

It's crucial to remember that, even while these groups can be more susceptible to problems, fifth disease is often a benign condition that heals on its own in healthy people. The symptoms often go away on their own and don't need any special medical attention.

It is recommended to seek early medical attention if there are concerns regarding possible exposure to fifth illness or if persons in high-risk populations get symptoms. It is especially important for expectant mothers to speak with their healthcare providers about how to monitor and manage any possible risks related to fifth disease.

CHAPTER THREE

Workplace and School Considerations

Some things to keep in mind when managing fifth disease (erythema infectiosum) in educational and professional environments include containing the virus and providing assistance for those who may be more susceptible to consequences. The following are important things to remember:

Educational Environments:

Consciousness and Instruction:

Teachers, administrators, and medical staff at schools should all be knowledgeable about the signs and ways in which the fifth disease spreads. Parents should also be provided with information.

Determining the Symptoms:

Instructors and other school personnel need to be on the lookout for signs of the fifth sickness, particularly the body's lacy rash and the recognizable "slapped cheek" rash. Those who are showing symptoms ought to be sent home with instructions to get help from a doctor.

Interaction with the parents:

Parents should be informed by schools about suspected cases of the fifth disease and encouraged to seek medical assistance for guidance and confirmation. The infectious nature of the virus and precautionary measures should be explained to parents.

Preventive actions:

Stress the importance of maintaining proper hygiene, such as frequent hand washing and respiratory etiquette (covering nose and mouth when sneezing or coughing). Promote hand sanitizer use, particularly for younger kids.

Separation of Affected Persons:

Until the contagious time has past, anyone exhibiting symptoms of the fifth sickness should be kept separate and returned home. This lessens the likelihood that the infection will spread across the school.

Expectant Instructors and Staff:

It is important to inform staff members and teachers who are expecting about the possible hazards related to fifth disease. It is important to share precautions, such as avoiding close contact with affected people.

Observation and Documentation:

Schools should keep an eye out for possible outbreaks and notify the local health authorities of any instances as needed. Appropriate preventative actions can be implemented with the aid of timely reporting.

Workplace Conditions:

Training Staff:

Workers should be informed by their employers about the signs and spread of the fifth disease.

This covers being aware of the infectious window and taking precautions.

Adaptable Work Schedules:

In order to lower the chance of the virus spreading throughout the company, take into consideration creating flexible work arrangements, such as remote work, if an employee is diagnosed with the fifth disease.

Hygienic habits

Encourage employees to exercise proper hygiene at work, such as frequent hand washing, hand sanitizer use, and respiratory etiquette. Posters and reminders should be displayed to promote these behaviors.

Talking with each other about symptoms:

When a fifth illness employee exhibits symptoms, they should be urged to notify their managers and get help right away. Employers might emphasize to staff members the value of timely reporting in order to stop the virus from spreading.

Employees that are expecting:

Employees who are expecting should be made aware of the possible hazards related to fifth disease. It is important to discuss precautions, like avoiding close contact with infected people, and accommodations might be taken into account.

Sanitizing and disinfecting:

In the workplace, frequent cleaning and disinfection of frequently touched surfaces can help lower the risk of transmission.

It's crucial to remember that people who exhibit fifth illness symptoms should consult a doctor right once, especially if they are pregnant or have weaker immune systems. In both business and educational environments, putting preventive measures into place and keeping lines of communication open can help create a safer and healthier atmosphere.

Long-Term Repercussions and Difficulties

Erythema infectiosum, often known as fifth disease, is typically a minor and self-limiting viral infection that resolves on its own for the majority of patients with no long-term problems. However, there may be related difficulties in particular people or situations. The following are possible fifth disease complications and long-term effects:

Joint Pain and Arthritis:

Arthritis and joint pain can occasionally be brought on by fifth illness, especially in adults. Joint pain may last for several weeks or months following the initial infection's cure. Women experience this more frequently than men do.

Problems in People with Haemolytic Disorders:

People who already suffer from hemolytic illnesses, like sickle cell anemia, may be more susceptible to consequences from fifth disease, which can include severe anemia.

Problems in Immunocompromised Persons:

Individuals who are immunocompromised, such as those receiving chemotherapy or living with HIV/AIDS, may have more severe and protracted symptoms. Anemia can result from parvovirus B19's impact on red blood cell formation.

Fetalis hydrops (in expectant mothers):

In rare instances, if a pregnant woman has fifth disease, there may be dangers to the developing fetus. It may result in hydrops fetalis, a condition in which the fetus has severe anemia. This may lead to miscarriage or stillbirth, as well as heart failure and other issues.

Prolonged Red Cell Hyperplasia:

Chronic red cell aplasia, a disorder in which the bone marrow is unable to generate enough red blood cells, has been linked to parvovirus B19. This is an uncommon consequence that is more frequently seen in those with underlying hematological disorders.

It is crucial to stress that the majority of people, especially healthy children, experience fifth disease as a self-limited illness and that severe complications are quite uncommon. Furthermore, while arthritis and joint discomfort might happen, they normally subside over time and are only brief.

In order to determine the possible hazards to the developing child, pregnant women who are exposed to the fifth disease or who exhibit symptoms should contact a doctor right away. Similar to this, those with weakened immune systems or underlying medical issues would need ongoing medical supervision.

Early medical action and appropriate cleanliness practices are two examples of preventive strategies that can help reduce the likelihood of fifth disease complications. For proper advice and evaluation, people should speak with healthcare professionals if they have concerns about possible exposure or symptoms.

Managing a viral infection such as fifth disease, or erythema infectiosum, can have a negative emotional and psychological impact, particularly on those who may be more susceptible to complications or experience symptoms for an extended period of time. The following are some methods to assist mental health and manage the difficulties brought on by the fifth disease:

Knowledge and Consciousness:

Anxiety can be reduced by being aware of the fifth disease's characteristics, typical symptoms, and chances of recovery. Those who receive trustworthy information from reliable sources and medical practitioners can better handle the emotional effects of their disease.

Looking for Assistance:

Talk to dependable family members, friends, or medical professionals about your worries and emotions. Having emotional support can help you deal with the anxiety and stress of being sick.

Getting Along with Others:

Make connections with those who have suffered from the fifth disease or related conditions. Online forums and support groups can offer a forum for exchanging knowledge, perspectives, and coping mechanisms.

Techniques for Relaxation and Mindfulness:

Utilize relaxation methods, mindfulness, or meditation to control stress and enhance emotional health. These methods can assist people in lowering their anxiety levels and helping them concentrate on the here and now.

Sustaining an Invigorating Lifestyle:

Make physical health a priority by leading a healthy lifestyle. Getting enough sleep, maintaining hydration, and eating a healthy diet all support resilience and general well-being throughout the healing process.

Recognizing Difficulties:

Concerns can be managed for those who are more likely to experience complications by being aware of the risks and talking about them with healthcare professionals. Having open lines of communication with medical experts might give comfort.

Communicating Feelings:

Give yourself permission to feel everything, including fear, grief, and irritation. Emotional expression can be achieved by journaling, painting, or speaking with a mental health professional.

Sustaining Social Relationships:

Maintain relationships with family and friends. In addition to providing emotional support, social ties can lessen feelings of loneliness experienced by patients.

Having Reasonable Expectations:

Understand that recovering from a fifth disease may require some time, particularly if joint pain or other issues are present. A positive outlook can be promoted by acknowledging accomplishments and having reasonable expectations.

Expert Guidance:

It may be helpful to seek out professional counseling or therapy if feelings of depression or anxiety do not go away. Mental health specialists can offer support during the healing process as well as coping mechanisms for emotional difficulties.

It's critical to customize coping mechanisms to meet the needs and preferences of each individual. Individuals may react differently to the emotional components of a medical condition, so it's important to seek professional assistance when necessary to promote emotional well-being. Keeping lines of communication open with medical professionals during the recuperation process can also aid with mental and physical issues.

CONCLUSION

In conclusion, the parvovirus B19 is the cause of the fifth disease, erythema infectiosum, which is often a minor and self-limiting viral infection. Pregnant women, those with compromised immune systems, and people with certain underlying medical disorders may be more susceptible to complications, even though the majority of cases end in minimal symptoms and full recovery.

The defining symptoms of the fifth disease are the lacy rash on the trunk and limbs and the characteristic "slapped cheek" rash on the face. The majority of the time, supportive care such as rest and fluids is adequate to manage the infection until it clears up.

Although they are uncommon, consequences can include severe anemia, joint discomfort, arthritis, and problems in pregnant women such hydrops fetalis. Managing fifth illness requires identifying possible dangers and obtaining medical assistance as soon as possible, particularly in high-risk populations.

Good hygiene habits and other preventive measures can help lower the chance of transmission, particularly in locations like workplaces and schools. Effective management involves communicating with healthcare providers, isolating affected persons during the contagious period, and recognizing symptoms early.

People and families who are coping with a fifth disease may feel anxious and stressed emotionally, particularly if there are unknowns or difficulties. Emotional well-being is influenced by exercising coping mechanisms, reaching out to people who have gone through similar experiences, and requesting assistance from medical professionals.

Maintaining a positive and knowledgeable mindset while being aware of the potential risks is crucial when managing fifth disease. Through education, obtaining the right medical advice, and taking care of their emotional health, people can effectively manage the effects of their disease and work toward a complete and healthy recovery.

THE END